THE TRAVELLER'S GUIDE
TO HOMOEOPATHY

by

PHYLLIS SPEIGHT

THE C. W. DANIEL COMPANY LIMITED
CHURCH PATH, SAFFRON WALDEN
ESSEX

First published in Great Britain by
The C. W. Daniel Company Limited
1 Church Path, Saffron Walden
Essex CB10 1JP, England

Reprinted 1993

ISBN 0 85207 212 0

The Random House Group Limited supports The Forest Stewardship
Council (FSC®), the leading international forest certification organisation.
Our books carrying the FSC label are printed on FSC® certified paper.
FSC is the only forest certification scheme endorsed by the leading
environmental organisations, including Greenpeace. Our
paper procurement policy can be found at
www.randomhouse.co.uk/environment

Printed and bound in Great Britain by Clays Ltd, St Ives PLC

CONTENTS

INTRODUCTION

Our mode of travel has been completely revolutionized during the last few decades.

Business men and politicians rush around the world and holiday makers are able to visit exotic places that were completely out of reach at the beginning of this century — all due to high speed aircraft.

Modern transport has, however, created additional hazards and because of the swiftness of travel we may not arrive at our destination with a clear head and comfortable body.

Various drugs are available to combat troubles caused by travel but there is a growing awareness that they can produce side-effects even if they can clear up the immediate problem.

Homoeopathy has much to offer in this field and in the majority of cases homoeopathic remedies are more effective than allopathic drugs. The additional advantage is that they have no side-effects whatsoever.

I very much hope that everyone who uses this small book will derive benefit from the information and that travelling will become enjoyable and free from anxieties.

Phyllis Speight

HOW TO USE THIS BOOK

This book has been written in order to provide the traveller with a simple guide to the homoeopathic treatment of many conditions that occur before, during and after a journey. It is suggested that the contents be studied to enable the reader to fully comprehend the scope of the work and thus be prepared to apply the appropriate treatment without delay.

It will be observed that injuries and some minor troubles can be overcome very simply. However, other ailments need more careful attention.

When dealing with troubles such as a stomach upset, headache, sleeplessness etc., the remedy which most closely matches the symptoms of the patient should be administered.

To assist in the selection of the correct remedy the symptoms should be **written down** under the following headings:-

LOCATION: The spot where there is an ache or pain (e.g., over the left eye; back of head etc., if a headache is being treated).

SENSATION: Describe exactly how it feels (e.g., aching, throbbing, sore, numb etc.).

MODALITIES: Anything that makes the trouble better or worse (e.g., heat, movement, weather, pressure etc.).

2

CAUSE: If known.

The section 'Characteristics and Modalities' has been compiled to simplify the identification of the appropriate remedy. A superficial study of homoeopathic remedies shows that many carry almost identical symptoms which, to the inexperienced prescriber, is confusing, but the characteristics and modalities are a key factor in the choice where two or more medicines cover much the same symptoms.

In this small book only the leading remedies have been given under each section, and they will be effective in the great majority of cases.

Unlike allopathic drugs, homoeopathic remedies are very sensitive and they should not be packed or carried near any strongly perfumed articles such as soaps, scents etc.

When taking homoeopathic remedies each pill or tablet should be placed under the tongue and allowed to dissolve. Do not wash down with water.

BEFORE THE JOURNEY

Many people suffer from 'nerves', anticipation and excitement before setting out on a journey, and this can happen before a holiday or business trip.

One of the following remedies should be helpful. It may be taken one or two days before leaving home, according to the severity of the symptoms.

ACONITE: There is acute anxiety and horrible fears — thoughts chase one another; forebodings with restlessness and impatience.
Great fear of flying.

ARGENTUM NITRICUM: Fearful and apprehensive before **any** ordeal: fear of heights, crowds, closed spaces, water.
Great anticipation.
Feels as though he/she can't get things done quickly enough.
All these thoughts cause diarrhoea.

GELSEMIUM: Emotional excitement; there is apprehension before any ordeal but those who need this remedy are quiet, subdued and trembling.
There is a fear of flying.

Remedies for the above mentioned conditions are needed in the 30th potency.

The dose should be 1 pill night and morning for one or two days before the journey. One dose on waking on the day of the journey and then as required for up to 3 more doses.

THE JOURNEY

DURING:—

ARGENTUM NITRICUM: Claustrophobic in a plane, or any vehicle — het-up, cannot keep still, very active.

COCCULUS: THE remedy for nausea, giddiness, faintness and loss of orientation.

GELSEMIUM: Nausea due to being nervous and tense. Claustrophobic and although het-up is silent and sits perfectly still.

NUX VOMICA: Acute headache over one eye, sometimes at the back of head, with nausea; tummy feels very queasy, cannot bear the thought of food.
Much retching and gagging.
Feels very cold and wants warmth.

PETROLEUM: Nausea and sickness due to inhaling exhaust fumes which can cause vomiting and heavy sweating.
There may be persistent nausea and an accumulation of water in the mouth.
Worse from petrol fumes; better for eating.

RHUS TOXICODENDRON: Air sickness; there is nausea and vomiting; extreme giddiness on trying to get up; severe frontal headache; no appetite, mouth very dry, very thirsty.

TABACUM: Nausea, giddiness and vomiting with icy coldness, and a sinking feeling. Worse from smell of tobacco smoke.

JUST BEFORE LANDING:—

BORAX: Fear of downward motion when plane begins to lose height; traveller can feel nauseated and may vomit.

PULSATILLA: Acute pain in ears when plane begins to lose height.

JET-LAG:—

ARNICA: Feeling of physical tiredness with aching muscles and limbs.

GELSEMIUM: Tiredness with heaviness of limbs.

The above mentioned remedies should be taken in the 6th or 12th potency, 1 pill at fifteen minute intervals for 3 or 4 doses if required, but if feeling better after the first dose or two do not repeat unless symptoms return.

For JET-LAG 1 pill of the indicated remedy hourly for 3 doses and then three hourly until symptoms disappear.

ACCIDENTS AND INJURIES

ARNICA: This is the first remedy that should be taken after any accident or injury because it not only deals with bruises of the soft (fleshy) parts, but it removes the shock which always follows any physical injury. It should be administered as quickly as possible.

One pill of the 200th potency will have a very quick effect. It may be repeated once or twice more if and when necessary.

CALENDULA: Is the most efficient healing agent which should be used immediately for abrasions from falls and accidents. The wound should be cleansed with cold water first and then a pad soaked in Calendula lotion (ten drops of the mother tincture (Ø) to a small wineglass of water applied. This should be kept moist by adding more lotion to the pad without removing it; healing usually takes place in record time.

HYPERICUM: For injuries to nerves — finger-ends, toes, the base of the spine (coccyx) and anywhere else where nerves are injured. The pain can be excruciating.

Children who get fingers jammed in doors gradually stop crying and can manage to smile again in a very short time if Hypericum is prescribed.

LEDUM: Is excellent for puncture wounds caused by any sharp object pushed into the flesh, e.g., splinter in the finger.

Ledum is needed when the wound feels cold and is better for cold applications.

Hypericum is helpful in similar circumstances if the wound is very painful and pains begin to shoot up the limb away from the wound.

Both these remedies act as anti-tetanus agents if tetanus (lockjaw) is likely, and symptoms agree.

RUTA: For sprains. Twisting an ankle or arm may wrench or damage ligaments or muscles causing much pain. After Arnica, Ruta will help especially if the injury is near a bone and the periosteum (bone covering) is damaged.

Bruised bones also respond well to Ruta.

RHUS TOXICODENDRON: Excellent for sprains. However, if the seat of the trouble feels cold and numb but better for cold applications and worse for warmth **Ledum** is the remedy. If the sprain is not serious and confined to the muscle there will be internal bruising and Arnica will probably clear up the trouble.

SYMPHYTUM: If a bone is broken, Arnica should be administered as soon as possible to help relieve the pain and remove the shock. Professional help will be needed for the bone to be set and then Symphytum should be given to help it knit together more quickly and reduce pain during the process.

One pill of the 30th potency night and morning for two weeks.

> The above mentioned remedies, with the exception of Arnica, Calendula, Symphytum, should be used in the 6th or 12th potency. One pill as often as every fifteen minutes for 3 doses if required but at longer intervals as soon as symptoms improve.

BACK AND NECK PROBLEMS

ANTIMONIUM TARTARICUM: Violent pains in sacro-lumbar region. The slightest effort to move is so painful it could cause retching and clammy sweat.
Worse in evening; from lying at night; from warmth; in cold damp weather.
Better sitting erect.

BRYONIA: Painful stiffness in nape of neck. Stitches and stiffness in small of back, brought on by changes in weather.
Worse from warmth; **any motion;** exertion; touch.
Better lying on painful side; pressure; rest.

GUAIACUM: Pain from head to neck. Aching in nape.
Stiff neck and sore shoulders.
Worse from motion; heat; cold wet weather; pressure; touch; from 6 p.m. to 4 a.m.
Better for external pressure.

KALI CARBONICUM: Great exhaustion, small of back feels weak. Burning in spine. Lumbago with sudden sharp pains extending up and down back and thighs.
Worse in cold weather; about 3 a.m.; lying on left and painful side.
Better in warm weather, though moist; during day, while moving about.

RHUS TOXICODENDRON: Pain and stiffness in small of back; better motion or lying on something hard. Also stiffness of nape of neck. Worse cold, wet weather and after rain; at night; during rest; when lying on back or right side.

Better warm dry weather; motion; walking; change of position; rubbing; warm applications; from stretching out limbs.

One pill of the 6th or 12th potency 3 times daily for a week or two, depending on the severity of the symptoms.

BLISTERS

CALENDULA ointment is helpful. Apply to blister; if not available bathe with a solution of Calendula Ø (mother tincture), ten drops in a small wineglass of water.

CAUSTICUM 12, one pill 3 times daily for a few days will also help.

BOILS AND CARBUNCLES

ANTHRACINUM: The 30th potency, night and morning, is excellent for septic inflammation. For boils and carbuncles when there is great burning and inflammation. It helps to clear up a succession of boils.
The eruption is bluish and often there is a black centre.

HEPAR SULPHURICUM: When there is a tendency to suppuration and great sensitivity to pain.

HYPERICUM: Mother tincture (Ø) for external application for both boils and carbuncles, especially when there is extensive laceration of tissues.

SILICA: The 6th potency, every three hours, helps to promote suppuration when the boil does not develop quickly.

TARENTULA CUBENSIS: Is most effective in both boils and carbuncles.
Sometimes a boil disappears before it really develops!
There is acute inflammation, stinging, throbbing and burning.

Unless otherwise stated 1 pill of the 6th or 12th potency should be taken every 3 hours for a few doses. As soon as improvement begins lengthen the time between doses and stop taking the remedy as soon as the condition clears up.

BURNS

URTICA URENS: Unless very severe, many burns will respond to this remedy when taken internally as well as being applied externally. For the latter a pad should be soaked in a solution of ten drops of mother tincture (Ø) in a wineglassful of water and applied to the burn; the pad should be kept damp by pouring a little of the solution on to it and, at the same time, one dose of the 30th potency taken as is necessary according to the severity of the burn. A dose may be taken as often as every 10 minutes to allay pain; but at longer intervals as soon as there is an improvement.

There is usually some shock with this type of injury, and a dose of Arnica 200 given immediately is recommended to overcome this trouble, or Aconite 200 if the patient is full of fear.

COLDS AND CHILLS

ACONITE: Should be taken immediately the first sneeze or shiver is felt.

Chills are often due to standing in a strong north or easterly gale whilst waiting for transport.

There is frequent sneezing with dropping of clear hot water from nostrils; there may be fever and thirst.

Patient is anxious, restless.

Worse from stuffy atmosphere; warm room.

Better in open air.

ARSENICUM ALBUM: Colds develop with every change of weather.

There is a thin watery, burning discharge; nose feels stopped up; much sneezing without any relief, or is stuffed up particularly at night.

Thirst for small amounts of water.

Patient is restless and anxious.

Worse in open air.

Better indoors; heat; warm drinks.

GELSEMIUM: Should be thought of where there is an influenza type of cold which often develops in warm, moist weather or when weather changes.

Sneezing; fullness at root of nose.

Discharge makes nostrils sore.

Chills run up and down spine; patient is hot and cold alternately and there is a heavy feeling in

head, eye-lids and limbs with tearing, tickling cough which is better near a fire.
Patient feels very tired.

NATRUM MURIATICUM: A heavy head cold with sneezing and very fluent running of the nose from one to three days, then the nose gets stopped up and discharge becomes like the white of an egg. The nose gets very sore inside. Cold sores around mouth.
It is said that this remedy is infallible for stopping a cold commencing with sneezing, if given quickly.

NUX VOMICA: Chills and colds from exposure to dry, cold winds; the patient cannot get warm even by the addition of extra clothes or sitting near an enormous fire.
There is much sneezing, the nose is stuffed up at night, streams in a warm room during the day.
Mouth dry.
Patient very irritable and snappy; nothing is right for him. He hates draughts. Better out of doors.

*One pill of the 6th or 12th potency should be given at half-hourly intervals at the **first signs** of a cold. Then 1 pill three hourly with longer periods between doses as symptoms improve.*

CONSTIPATION

ALUMINA: When caused by unusual food and eating at different times from the normal hours.

Inactivity of rectum.

Great straining to pass even a soft stool.

No desire for, and no ability to pass, stool, with large accumulation.

Rectum seems paralysed.

BRYONIA: No desire, stool unsatisfactory after much straining; stools hard, dark, dry, as if burnt. Very large.

Abdomen distended, there is rumbling with cutting pains, yet obstinate constipation.

Thirst for long drinks.

Patient is irritable.

NUX VOMICA: Constant urging to stool which never comes, or a small stool comes with difficulty and a feeling that the evacuation is incomplete.

Bloated sensation.

Trouble often caused by over-eating and over-drinking.

Patient feels chilly and is irritable.

OPIUM: Obstinate constipation; no desire to go to stool.

Faeces protrude and recede.

There can be violent pain in the rectum.

One pill of the 6th or 12th potency three times daily for a week or two should help providing symptoms agree.

CRAMP

ARNICA: Cramping pains in calves of legs caused by fatigue.

CUPRUM: Cramps in palms of hands, calves of legs, soles of feet.
Contraction of muscles and tendons — very painful.

NUX VOMICA: Cramp occurs in calves of legs and soles of feet at night only.
Patient wants to stretch the feet.

LEDUM: Has cleared up many cases of cramp when the cause is unknown — it is well-worth trying if there are no indications for one of the above-mentioned remedies.

One pill of the 6th or 12th potency should be taken at ten minute intervals for up to 3 doses. If the trouble has not completely disappeared take a few more doses at half hourly intervals.

DIARRHOEA

ACONITE: Diarrhoea brought on by exposure to dry cold wind, or the result of a fright.

ARSENICUM ALBUM: When diarrhoea and vomiting occur together, especially in gastro-enteritis, or when food poisoning is suspected. Patient is very cold, very restless, irritable and exhausted.
There is a desire for hot drinks.

CHINA (Cinchona): Painless diarrhoea, undigested, frothy, yellow; after fruit, milk, beer, and in hot weather, with much flatulence. Patient feels very weak.
Can occur after a summer chill.
This remedy should be given after any loss of fluids.

COLOCYNTH: Agonising pain in abdomen causing patient to bend double, diarrhoea recurring after eating or drinking.
Trouble is often caused by anger.

DULCAMARA: Diarrhoea from suddenly feeling chilled when hot, or from getting cold and wet.

NUX VOMICA: Diarrhoea after a party, after eating and/or drinking too much; sometimes alternating with constipation.
Worse in morning.

One pill of the 6th or 12th potency at two hourly intervals — leave a longer gap between doses as soon as symptoms improve.

Professional advice must be sought if symptoms do not improve.

EAR TROUBLES

ACONITE: Sudden earache after exposure to cold winds or to very cold weather.
Ear red, hot, painful; better for warm applications.
Pain may be violent.
Sometimes better for local heat.

BELLADONNA: Sudden onset, particularly when right ear is affected.
Digging, throbbing pain; face flushed; red, hot, dry burning skin. Pain worse least jar. Better for heat.
Patient restless.
Very little thirst.

CHAMOMILLA: Patient very sensitive to pain which makes him/her irritable.
Pain is worse from warm applications.
Children often have one red, hot cheek, the other pale and cold with earache; they are very fretful.

COCA: Noises in ears when in high altitudes.

FERRUM PHOSPHORICUM: The most commonly indicated remedy in the very early stages, when symptoms are not very distinctive.
First stages of inflammation such as occur in ear infection.

MAGNESIUM PHOSPHORICUM: Earache is usually from exposure to cold winds rather than an actual infection.

The right ear is mostly affected.

Pain worse washing in cold water.

Better for warmth.

PULSATILLA: Redness and swelling of external ear.

Severe throbbing pain and ears feel stopped up.

Trouble brought on by becoming chilled and getting wet.

There may be fever.

Pain is worse for warmth and from becoming overheated. Worse in evenings and at night.

Patient craves fresh air; wants attention and company; is tearful.

Professional advice must be sought if symptoms do not improve within a reasonable time.

One pill of the 6th or 12th potency every two hours for 3 doses, then three hourly for the rest of the day followed by a dose 3 times daily until the symptoms clear up; if symptoms are very acute at onset 1 pill every fifteen minutes for up to 3 doses.

EYE TROUBLES

Injuries to eyes often need attention from a doctor whose help should be sought.

ARNICA: Administer immediately in any injury, even before seeking expert advice.
Injuries from grit and other foreign bodies will respond to this remedy.
One dose of the 30th potency as soon as possible.

CALENDULA: As a temporary measure in an injury apply a pad soaked in a lotion of 10 drops of mother tincture (Ø) in a wineglassful of water.

EUPHRASIA: Pain after a foreign body has been removed will be helped by bathing with a lotion of 10 drops of mother tincture (Ø) in a wineglassful of warm water. An eyebath is helpful.

HYPERICUM: For dust or foreign body in eye bathe with a lotion of 10 drops of mother tincture (Ø) in a wineglassful of water.
If a foreign body is deeply embedded seek professional advice but, meanwhile, insert a drop of Castor Oil then cover with a large pad.

LEDUM: Almost a specific for a 'black eye' if it feels better for cool applications.

RUTA: An excellent remedy for eyestrain caused by too much reading, staring or concentrating for too long on an object.

One pill of the 6th or 12th potency three times daily for up to two weeks.

SYMPHYTUM: Pain in eyeball and often in surrounding bone, caused by a blow from a ball or stone.

The dose for Ledum and Symphytum is 1 pill of the 6th or 12th potency every fifteen minutes for up to 3 doses and then less frequently as the pain subsides.

FAINTING

There are a number of causes — fatigue, insufficient food, lack of fresh air, sudden emotion, tight clothing, are just a few.

When fainting occurs the patient should be put down flat and clothing loosened, especially round the waist and neck.

Give the patient plenty of air.

Select one of the following remedies according to the symptoms and place 1 pill, a few granules or a drop of the tincture inside the lower lip or under the tongue.

Fainting from lack of air (hot, stuffy room) **Pulsatilla**.

Fainting from loss of blood **China**.

Fainting from the sight of blood **Nux vomica**.

Fainting from pain **Aconite** or **Chamomilla**.

Fainting from fatigue **Arnica**.

Fainting from climbing mountains **Coca**.

Fainting from nervous anticipation, fear **Gelsemium**.

Fainting from excitement **Coffea**.

Use in the 6th or 12th potency and the dose may be repeated within a few minutes, if necessary.

FEET AND LEG PROBLEMS

ANTIMONIUM CRUDUM: For cracked heels with hard skin, or if the feet become tender and hard skin develops.

One pill of the 6th or 12th potency 3 times daily for a week or two.

APIS: Swelling and puffiness of feet and ankles.
Worse heat.

One pill of the 6th or 12th potency 3 times daily for one week.

ARNICA: Tired and fatigued feet and legs from exertion, over-walking, climbing, etc. Soak the feet and, if necessary the body, in a bath of hot water to which has been added a few drops of Arnica mother tincture (Ø); a full bath should have a few more drops. It is very soothing.
A dose of Arnica 200 is beneficial.

CALENDULA: If feet become blistered Calendula cream or ointment rubbed in gently will be of great help.

FOOD POISONING

ACONITE: If there are symptoms of poisoning with restless tossing and turning plus great fear.

ARSENICUM ALBUM: Ptomaine poisoning. Severe vomiting and diarrhoea with great exhaustion and restlessness.

CARBO VEGETABILIS: Poisoning from bad fish with marked collapse, and desire to be fanned as patient cannot get enough air.

PULSATILLA: Poisoning from bad fish or meat. There is a craving for fresh air; very rarely any thirst.

URTICA URENS: Poisoning from eating shellfish. Itching blotches with burning heat.

VERATRUM ALBUM: Poisoning with severe vomiting and diarrhoea, collapse and cold sweat on forehead.

One pill of the 6th or 12th potency at fifteen minute intervals for up to 3 doses, then less frequently until symptoms subside.

FROST-BITE

In very cold regions, for instance in snowy, mountainous country, exposed parts, nose, ears, toes and fingers may get frost bitten. All feeling is lost at first, then parts become white and later congested and bluish in colour.

The first important action is to rub snow into the affected part which will stimulate the contracted blood vessels and cause them to dilate and bring back circulation.

After that the patient should have hot drinks — coffee, tea or soup, and if exhausted he should be put into a warm bed.

FERRUM PHOSPHORICUM: Would supplement the above mentioned measures.

CHILBLAINS (minor frost-bite)

TAMUS COMMUNIS: The mother tincture (Ø) applied externally is usually most helpful.

CALENDULA: Where broken apply the mother tincture (Ø) instead of Tamus; or use Calendula ointment.

The following should be given internally:-

AGARICUS: Chilblains of feet, toes, hands. Worse for cold.
Better for warmth.

HEPAR SULPHURICUM: Suppurating, very painful chilblains which are tender to touch.

PULSATILLA: Inflamed, intensely itching, purple chilblains that are worse for heat, a warm room, in a hot bed, sitting in front of a fire.

RHUS TOXICODENDRON: Much burning and intense itching with dark red inflammation which is covered with blisters.
Worse in damp-cold.

One pill of the 6th or 12th potency at three hourly intervals for 3 doses and then three times daily until cured.

HEADACHES
AND SUNSTROKE

In cases of sunstroke the temperature should be reduced by cold sponging in a cool or shady spot or room.

ARNICA: If brought on by a fall or injury.
Head feels hot and body cold.
There may be chronic giddiness, objects whirl around, especially when walking.
Violent headaches in children with vomiting from anticipation and excitement.
Child very restless.

BELLADONNA: Sunstroke — throbbing in head and arteries with rush of blood to head after being exposed to too much sun; face red and flushed, pupils dilated.
Bounding pulse, burning, hot dry skin with delirium.
Headache after having hair cut or shampooed and then going out into cold air.

BRYONIA: When headache is caused by constipation, it can feel bursting and settles in the back of the neck.
Very bad headache after too much sun, with nausea.
Worse on movement and sitting up.

COCA: Headache caused by high altitudes — climbing mountains.

Headache with giddiness, preceded by flashes of light.

Band-like feeling across forehead.

COCCULUS: Headaches at back of head and nape of neck when riding in a car or any vehicle, with giddiness and nausea.

Opening and shutting sensation.

GELSEMIUM: Violent hammering pains in head (often accompanied by diarrhoea) in children who suffer from anticipation, fear and the effects of sudden surprises which make them feel weak, faint and exhausted.

GLONOINE: Headaches from the effects of too much sun.

There is a sense of confusion with dizziness.

Throbbing, bursting sensation, head feels heavy.

Cannot bear any heat around head.

Flushed face and sweaty skin.

Sun headaches increase and decrease with the sun.

Patient very irritable.

Better from uncovering head in cool and shade.

KALI PHOSPHORICUM: Occipital (back of head and neck) headache from fatigue, pain better after rising, with weary, all gone sensation in stomach.

Better from gentle motion.

NUX VOMICA: Headache from loss of sleep after eating and drinking too much — wakes up feeling awful — the morning after the night before.

Head feels heavy.

Constipation makes headache worse.

PULSATILLA: Frontal headache and/or pressure on top of head, from eating too much rich, greasy, fatty food or ice cream.

33

Better in open air and walking slowly in the cool.

One pill of the 6th or 12th potency two or three hourly according to the severity of the headache for up to 3 doses, then less often. In cases of sunstroke, 1 pill at half-hourly intervals for up to 3 doses and then less often.

NOSE BLEED

ARNICA: Given at once will stop bleeding if caused by an injury or blow.

PHOSPHORUS: For profuse bleeding, sometimes from a broken blood vessel after blowing vigorously.

FERRUM PHOSPHORICUM: May be taken if either of the above mentioned is not available.

One pill of the 12th potency every few minutes until improvement, then less frequently.

SLEEPLESSNESS

ACONITE: Restless sleep, tossing about.
Starts up in sleep.
Insomnia of the old.

ARNICA: Unable to sleep through being over-tired, physically or mentally.
Bed feels too hard; must keep moving, trying to get comfortable.

ARSENICUM ALBUM: Disturbed, anxious, restless sleep.
Dreams are full of fear.
Must sleep on several pillows.
Is so restless, has to get up and walk around.
Worse after midnight.

COFFEA: Cannot sleep because of mental activity, thoughts go round and round.
There is nervous excitability.
Often sleeps until 3 a.m. and then cannot get off again; only dozes.

GELSEMIUM: Cannot sleep because of exhaustion; or of uncontrollable thinking; also from nervous irritation.

NUX VOMICA: Sleepless after much mental work and strain, or from eating or drinking too much.
Wakes up at about 3 a.m. then goes to sleep much later and is cross and unrefreshed when it is time to get up.

One pill of the 12th or 30th potency on going to bed. May be repeated half to one hour later, if necessary.

STINGS AND BITES

APIS: Stings from insects when there is swelling and puffiness, redness of the skin and stinging pains with soreness.
There is intolerance of heat and the slightest touch.
Worse in the afternoon.

HYPERICUM: For all stings from insects if the pain shoots up the limb, away from the wound.

LEDUM: For all stings if the wound feels cold and is better for cold applications.
If allergic to stings **Ledum** should be taken daily whilst the danger is around.
  Insect bites should be treated with the above mentioned remedies — the symptoms must be matched.

One pill of the 6th or 12th potency at fifteen or thirty minute intervals for up to 3 doses, then at longer intervals.

SNAKE BITES If the venom is known give the following:—

NAJA for cobra.
VIPERA for adder.
LACHESIS for Surukuku (South American).
CROTALUS HORRIDUS for rattlesnake.
ELAPS CORALLINUS for coral snake (Brazilian).

Potency and dosage as above.

All snake bites should be treated with a local application of Permanganate of Potash and strong coffee to drink. A doctor should be called.

BITES FROM SPIDERS If the spider is identified the following remedy should be taken:—

LATRODECTUS MACTANS for Black Widow.
TARENTULA HISPANICA for Tarentula.
LATRODECTUS HASSELTI for Black Spider (Australian — New South Wales).

Potency and dosage as above.

DOG BITES can be dangerous where there is risk of rabies.

HYDROPHOBINUM 30 should be given daily, a dose on rising, and this should be supplemented by **Ledum** 30, a dose at night, over a long period where there is any possibility of rabies.
Professional help should be obtained.

STOMACH TROUBLES

ARSENICUM ALBUM: Burning pains in stomach after eating ice-cream, melon, watery fruit, or drinking ice-cold water.

There may be nausea and vomiting.

Everything that enters the stomach burns or is vomited.

Patient is fearful and restless.

BRYONIA: Violent pains in abdomen, with severe vomiting.

Cannot keep anything down and even though thirsty cold water will return as soon as it enters the stomach.

Patient wants to keep perfectly still, nausea and vomiting come on as soon as the head is raised or he tries to sit up.

Stomach pains better for hot applications.

Symptoms brought on by over-eating, rich food, cabbage, cheese, new bread, ice cream.

These troubles could also indicate the first stage of appendicitis so if the trouble does not respond to the remedy quickly a doctor should be called.

CARBO VEGETABILIS: Acute indigestion after eating pork, rich food, excess of rancid fat.

There is an accumulation of wind and distension of stomach; everything turns to wind, patient is always belching which gives temporary relief.

There is much anxiety and restlessness with distension, mainly on lying down at night.

Worse lying down.

Better sitting up and by loud eructations.

CHINA: Indigestion and colic after excess of fruit, eating cabbage, raw vegetables, pickles, flatulent food, and drinking too much tea.

Stomach is bloated and distended with constant belching which does not relieve.

Diarrhoea after eating, rumbling in abdomen and the expulsion of quantities of wind from the bowels.

Stools painless, yellow.

NUX VOMICA: Clears up symptoms of a common bilious attack coming on after exposure to cold, dry winds or draughts; after eating too much rich food and/or drinking too much alcohol, followed by strong coffee.

There is heaviness and a feeling of a weight in the stomach and chest a couple of hours after a meal and a general liverish feeling, cold, nausea and sometimes vomiting; skin and eyes look yellowish.

Patient is very irritable and snappy. Often takes laxatives.

Always feels better if he is sick.

PULSATILLA: Acute gastric disturbances after eating pork, pastry, ice-cream, too much rich, greasy food.

There is nausea, bloating of the stomach, colicky pains, belching of rancid food; mouth is slimy or dry, without thirst; a bad taste.

Cannot lie still with gastric and bowel symptoms.

Better in fresh air.

One pill of the 6th or 12th potency hourly

for 3 doses, then three hourly for the remainder of the day. Subsequently 1 pill 3 times daily until improvement.

MATERIA MEDICA

ACONITE

Characteristics:
Fear, anxiety, physical and mental restlessness.
Fright — Aconite has a calming effect.
The sudden beginning of an acute illness with fever, anxiety, restlessness and fear.
Fearful of the future, of death, there are so many fears.
Can vomit with fear.
There is much tension.
Complaints caused by exposure to dry cold winds and weather.

Modalities:
Worse: Warm room; around midnight; cold dry winds.
Better: Open air.

AGARICUS

Characteristics:
Jerking, twitching, trembling.
Sensation as if pierced by needles of ice.
Violent bearing down pains.
Symptoms appear diagonally, e.g. right arm and left leg.

Modalities:

Worse: Open cold air; in cold weather; before a thunder-storm; after eating.
Better: Moving about slowly.

ALUMINA

Characteristics:
Hasty, hurried, time passes too slowly.
Variable mood, better as day advances.
Dryness of mucous membranes.
Sluggish functions.
Abnormal cravings for chalk, charcoal, coffee grounds, indigestible things.

Modalities:
Worse: Morning; warm room.
Better: Open air and damp weather.

ANTHRACINUM

A nosode.

ANTIMONIUM CRUDUM

Characteristics:
Thickly coated white, very white tongue.
Derangements from overloading the stomach, especially with fat foods, nausea.
Finger nails grow in splits with horny spots.
Corns and callosities on soles of feet.
Child cannot bear to be looked at.
Fitful, cross.
Feverish conditions at night.
Cannot bear heat of sun.
Exhausted in warm weather.

Modalities:
Worse: Heat and heat of sun and radiated heat; cold bathing.

ANTIMONIUM TARTARICUM

Characteristics:
Great weakness, lassitude.

Drowsiness, debility and sweat.

Sleepiness or sleeplessness.

Great accumulation of mucus in air passages with much rattling and inability to raise it.

Nausea, vomiting, with loss of appetite.

Pallor. Pale sunken face.

Lack of thirst.

Irritability.

Modalities:
Worse: In evening; lying down at night; from warmth; in damp, cold weather.

Better: Sitting erect; from bringing up wind and expectoration.

APIS MELLIFICA

Characteristics:
Jealous and suspicious.

Whining; tearfulness.

Awkward, often drops things.

Constricted sensations.

Oedema.

Pains stinging and burning.

Alternately dry and hot or perspiring.

Thirstlessness; sweats without thirst.

Cannot stand heat; warm room, hot bath.

Modalities:
Worse: Heat in any form; pressure; late afternoon; after sleeping; in closed and heated rooms.

Better: In open air; uncovering; cold bathing.

ARGENTUM NITRICUM

Characteristics:
Fear, anxiety, apprehension regarding future events.

Funks examinations.

Fears failure. Tummy turns over.

Irrational thoughts and imaginations.

Impulsive, does things in a hurry, walks fast.

Claustrophobia.

Looking from heights causes giddiness, looking up at high buildings also causes trouble.

When in a theatre or other gathering seeks a seat which will enable him to make a quick exit or escape.

Dreads crowds.

Irresistible desire for sugar and sweet things which aggravate and cause diarrhoea.

Worse heat, feeling of suffocation in a warm room, wants cold air.

Modalities:

Worse: Warmth in any form; at night; from cold food; sweets; after eating; at menstrual period; from emotions; left side.

Better: From eructations; fresh air; cold; pressure.

ARNICA MONTANA

Characteristics

In serious illness says there is nothing the matter with him/her.

After traumatic injuries.

Sore, lame, bruised feeling.

Modalities:

Worse: Least touch; motion; rest; wine; damp cold.

Better: Lying down or head low.

ARSENICUM ALBUM

Characteristics:

Great anguish and restlessness.

Fear, fright and worry.

Prostration yet marked restlessness from anxiety making patient change places constantly.

Great exhaustion after slightest exertion.

Fastidious, hates disorder.

Burning pains better by heat but patient always wants the head kept cool.

Burning discharges.

Great thirst for small quantities at frequent intervals.

Modalities:

Worse: Cold air; wet weather; cold drinks; cold applications; night, after midnight, 1 a.m. to 3 a.m.

Better: Warmth (except head). Loves and craves heat.

BELLADONNA

Characteristics:

Heat, redness, throbbing, burning violent.

Acute local inflammations with sudden onset.

Fevers with dry, hot, burning skin, heat can be felt before hand touches it.

Very red flushed face.

Pupils dilated.

Sudden rise in temperature.

Restlessness from excitement.

Mental states which can go on to delirium.

Throbbing in head.

Modalities:

Worse: Touch, jar; noise; draught; after noon; lying down.

Better: Being semi-erect.

BORAX

Characteristics:

Dread of downward motion in nearly all complaints, which brings anxiety.

Very nervous and frightened.
Sensitive to sudden noise.

Modalities:
Worse: Warm weather.
Better: Cold weather.

BRYONIA

Characteristics:
Complaints develop slowly.
Great irritability. Don't cross a Bryonia patient,
it makes him/her worse.
Excessive thirst for copious draughts at long
intervals.
Stitching and tearing pains which are worse for
movement and better for rest.
Dryness of mucous membranes from lips to
rectum.
Faintness when head is raised (sitting up in
bed).

Modalities:
Worse: Warmth; slightest motion; eating; hot
weather; exertion; touch; cannot sit up, is faint
and sick.
Better: Lying on painful side; pressure; rest;
cold things.

COCA

Characteristics:
Palpitation; breathlessness; anxiety and
insomnia from mountain climbing.

Modalities:
Worse: Ascending high altitudes.
Better: From wine; riding; quick motion in
open air.

CHAMOMILLA

Characteristics:
Frantic, irritability — cannot bear it — whatever it may be!
Impatient, over-sensitive.
Whining restlessness; impatient, snappish.
Is bad tempered when he (she) cannot get what he wants.
Inability to control temper.

Modalities:
Worse: Heat; anger; open air; wind; at night.
Better: Warm, wet weather; from being carried (children).

CHINA (CINCHONA)

Characteristics:
Debility and complaints after excessive loss of fluids; bleeding; periods; diarrhoea.
Haemorrhage can be profuse with fainting.
Periodical affections, especially every other day.

Modalities:
Worse: Slightest touch; draught of air; loss of vital fluids; at night; after eating.
Better: Hard pressure on painful part; open air; warmth.

COCCULUS

Characteristics:
Extreme irritability of nervous system.
Cannot bear contradiction.
Profound sadness.
Effects of night-watching.
Sensation of hollowness — emptiness.

Time passes too quickly. Slowness in thinking.
Worse after an emotional disturbance.
Sensitive to jolt and cold air.

Modalities:
Worse: Eating; after loss of sleep; open air;
smoking; riding in a vehicle; swimming; touch;
noise; jar; afternoon; menstrual periods and
after emotional disturbances.

COFFEA

Characteristics:
Extreme sensitiveness. Unusual activity of mind
and body. Intolerance of pain.

Modalities:
Worse: Excessive emotions including joy;
narcotics; strong odours; noise; open air; cold;
night.
Better: Warmth; from lying down; holding ice
in mouth.

COLOCYNTH

Characteristics:
Agonizing pain in abdomen causing patient to
bend double.

Modalities:
Worse: From anger and indignation.
Better: Doubling up; hard pressure; warmth;
lying with head bent forward.

CUPRUM METALLICUM

Characteristics:
Spasmodic affections; cramps; violent con-
tractive and intermitting pain.

Modalities:

Worse: Before menses; from vomiting; contact.
Better: During perspiration; drinking cold water.

DULCAMARA

Characteristics:
Ailments from effects of damp weather.
After exposure to wet and hot days and cold nights.

Modalities:
Worse: Night; from cold in general; damp rainy weather.
Better: From moving about; external warmth.

EUPHRASIA

Characteristics:
Inflammation of conjunctival membrane producing profuse lachrymation.

Modalities:
Worse: Evening; indoors; warmth; south winds; light.
Better: In dark.

FERRUM PHOSPHORICUM

Characteristics:
Remedy for nervous, sensitive, anaemic patients.
Susceptibility to chest troubles.
For the first stage of all febrile disturbances where there are no other indications.

Modalities:
Worse: At night and 4 to 6 a.m.; touch; jar; motion; right side.
Better: Cold applications.

GELSEMIUM

Characteristics:
Affects more the nerves of motion, causing muscular prostration and varying degrees of motor paralysis.

Dizziness, drowsiness, dullness, trembling.

Tiredness, limbs feel tired; eyelids feel heavy.

Fearful; terrors of anticipation.

Apathy regarding illness.

Modalities:
Worse: Damp weather; emotion; excitement; bad news; 10 a.m.

Better: Bending forward; open air; continued motion. Headache is relieved by profuse urination.

GLONOINE

Characteristics:
Congestion of head.

Surging of blood to head and heart.

Sensation of pulsation throughout the body.

Pulsating pains.

Modalities:
Worse: In the sun; exposure to sun's rays; gas or open fire; jar; stooping; having hair cut; peaches; stimulants; lying down; from 6 a.m. to noon; left side.

GUAIACUM

Characteristics:
Action on fibrous tissue.

Feeling that he must stretch.

Contraction of limbs, stiffness.

Modalities:
Worse: From motion; heat; cold, wet weather; pressure; touch; from 6 p.m. to 4 a.m.

Better: External pressure.

HEPAR SULPHURICUM

Characteristics:
Hypersensitive. Irritable. Impetuous.
General sensitivity to all impressions, the slightest cause irritates.
Very sensitive to pain.
Feels as if wind is blowing on to some part.
Tendency to suppurations.
Sweats easily on slight exertion.

Modalities:
Worse: Dry cold wind; cool air; slightest draught.
Better: Damp weather; warmth; wrapped up head; after eating.

HYPERICUM

Characteristics:
Injury to nerves.
Puncture wounds.
Relieves pain after operations.

Modalities:
Worse: In cold; dampness; in fog; in close room; least exposure; touch.
Better: Bending head backward.

KALI CARBONICUM

Characteristics:
Very irritable.
Anxiety felt in the stomach.
Hypersensitive to pain, noise and touch.
All pains are sharp; cutting.
Stitches may be felt in any part of the body.
Intolerance of cold weather.

Modalities:
Worse: From soup and coffee; at 3 a.m.; lying on left and painful side.
Better: Warm, moist weather; moving about.

KALI PHOSPHORICUM

Characteristics:
Conditions arising from lack of nerve power.
Prostration.
Anxiety, nervous dread; lethargy.
Slightest labour seems a heavy task.
Night terrors.

Modalities:
Worse: Excitement; worry; mental and physical exertion; eating; cold; early morning.
Better: Warmth; rest; nourishment.

LEDUM

Characteristics:
There is a general lack of animal heat yet heat of bed is intolerable.
Punctured wounds (bites) if wounded parts are cold.
Tetanus with twitching of muscles near wound and if wound is cold and feels better by cold.

Modalities:
Worse: At night and from heat of bed.
Better: From cold; putting feet in cold water.

MAGNESIA PHOSPHORICA

Characteristics:
Anti-spasmodic remedy.
Cramps.
Neuralgic pains relieved by warmth.
Tired, languid, exhausted patients.

Modalities:
Worse: Right side; cold; touch; at night.
Better: Warmth; bending double; pressure; friction.

NATRUM MURIATICUM

Characteristics:
Ill effects of grief, fright, anger.
Consolation aggravates; wants to be alone to cry.
Depressed; moody.
Very irritable.
Great weakness and weariness.
All mucous membranes dry.
Craves salt.
Very thirsty.

Modalities:
Worse: Noise; music; warm room; consolation; sea-shore (can be better sea-shore); heat and cold.
Better: Open air; cold bathing.

PETROLEUM

Characteristics:
Ailments from riding in cars, ships or planes.
Ailments worse during winter.
Diarrhoea only during daytime.
Tips of fingers rough, cracked, fissured every winter.

Modalities:
Worse: Dampness; before and during thunder-storms; from riding in vehicles; motion; in winter; from mental states.
Better: Warm air; lying with head high; dry weather.

PHOSPHORUS

Characteristics:
Extremely sensitive.
Fearful of thunder-storms; being alone; of the dark; disease; death.

Very affectionate; they need it and give it, yet there can be an indifference.

Desire to be rubbed.

Much weakness and trembling.

Burning pains.

Haemorrhages bright and freely flowing.

Thirst for cold drinks which are vomited as soon as they become warm.

Modalities:

Worse: Physical or mental exertion; twilight; warm food or drink; from getting wet in hot weather; change of weather; evening; lying on painful side.

Better: Heat (everywhere except in stomach and head).

Dr. Margaret Tyler says: 'Phosphorus complaints are worse from cold and cold weather, better from heat and warm applications, except for the complaints of head and stomach, which are ameliorated from cold.'

PULSATILLA

Characteristics:

The temperament is mild and gentle but anger can appear, and irritability.

Tears come very easily; inclined to silent grief.

Conscientious, hates to be hustled.

Loves sympathy and fuss.

Changeable in everything; in disposition (like an April shower and sunshine).

Pains wander from joint to joint; no two stools are alike, etc.

Pulsatilla feels the heat; they must have air, it makes them feel much better.

Cannot eat fat, rich food, it makes them feel sick.

Thirstless, even with a fever.

Modalities:

Worse: Warm room; warm applications. Cannot bear heat in any form.

Better: Cool open air; walking slowly in open air but pains of Pulsatilla are accompanied by chilliness.

RHUS TOXICODENDRON

Characteristics:

Extremely restless with continued change of position.

Great apprehension at night, cannot remain in bed.

Tearing pains.

Red triangle at tip of tongue.

Modalities:

Worse: During sleep; cold, wet rainy weather; after rain; during rest especially at night; cold air; getting wet.

Better: Warm, dry weather; motion; walking; change of position; rubbing; warm applications; from stretching the limbs.

RUTA GRAVEOLENS

Characteristics:

Acts on periosteum; complaints from straining flexor tendons especially.

Bruised feeling.

Intense lassitude, weakness and despair.

Modalities:

Worse: Over exertion; lying down; from cold, wet weather.

Better: Warmth; rubbing.

SILICA

Characteristics:

Want of grit — moral and physical.

Yielding, faint-hearted, anxious.
Very sensitive to all impressions.
Easily irritated over trifles; touchy and self-willed.
Fixed ideas.
Intolerance of alcohol.
Suppurative processes.
Under-nourished from imperfect assimilation.
Feels the cold.

Modalities:
Worse: Morning; uncovering; damp.
Better: Warmth; wrapping up head; in the summer; in wet or humid weather.

SYMPHYTUM

Characteristics:
Injuries to sinews, tendons and periosteum.
Acts on joints generally.
Wounds penetrating to the perineum and bones and non-union of fractures.
Pricking pain.

TABACUM

Characteristics:
Nausea, giddiness, death-like pallor, vomiting, icy-coldness; sweat with intermittent pulse.
Chills with cold sweat.

Modalities:
Worse: Opening eyes; evening; extremes of heat and cold.
Better: Uncovering; open, fresh air.

TARENTULA CUBENSIS

Characteristics:
Septic conditions.

Severe inflammation and pain.
Skin purple hue.

Modalities:
Worse: At night.

URTICA URENS

Characteristics:
Pains stinging and itching.

Modalities:
Worse: From snow-air; water; cool moist air;
touch.